# Contents

# COLLOIDAL SILVER - THE NATURAL ANTIBIOTIC

## THE HOLISTIC ALTERNATIVE TO ANTIBIOTICS NEW DISCOVERED

MARCUS D. ADAMS

# ONE

## COLLOIDAL SILVER

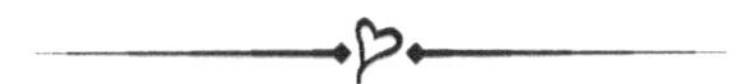

Through the years, the medical capabilities of colloidal silver have been growing undeniably. This solution has been in existence for centuries. Lethal bacteria, such as anthrax and HIV, and antibiotic-resistant organisms, like staph and pseudomonas, are said to be destroyed by colloidal silver. Risks of using colloidal silver are minimal compared to many modern drugs, and side effects are very rare.

Colloidal silver has also been used for curing water. In fact, the National Aeronautics and Space Administration has used colloidal silver as a means to purify water in space, avoiding the use of chlorine.

Despite the many uses of colloidal silver, Food and Drug Administration of the United States has not lifted the ban it imposed a few years back. There have been no pharmaceutical companies willing to come out and support the funding of a patented product involving colloidal silver. Studies have shown that profit margins for developing a colloidal silver product would not be worthwhile for companies. Funding the research for continuous development of the product would be too costly. And there have been various colloidal silver generators developed that could allow you to create your own at home.

Furthermore, there are no proven drug effects involving the use of silver, so it is very difficult to developing a guideline for proper use of colloidal silver. It is unknown how the body actually reacts to the silver at a given dosage.

To illustrate this, let's say you have a headache. You know you can take two aspirins and you will be relieved. But with colloidal silver, there is no telling how much you need to take. For some people, one teaspoon is enough. But for others, many ounces in a span of 45 minutes to hours or even days are needed just to relieve a common sore throat, for example. The dosage of intake varies from one person to another, even from the same batch

# TWO

# WHAT IS COLLOIDAL SILVER

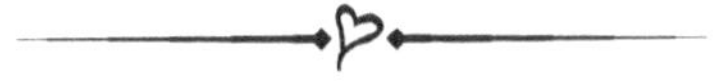

Colloidal silver is a completely natural, liquid, broad-spectrum infection-fighting agent found in almost every health food store in North America. It is made through a simple electromagnetic process that pulls microscopic particles of silver from a larger piece of pure silver immersed in water. These tiny silver particles are held in suspension in the resulting solution by the electric charge on each atom. When ingested, they travel throughout your body like any other mineral before being excreted through your normal channels of elimination. But as they come into contact with pockets of infection in your body, they kill virtually every pathogenic microorganism in the vicinity, bringing about rapid healing.

100 Year Medical History - The simple process for producing colloidal silver was developed shortly after Edison harnessed electricity in 1892. It was then used for decades

by doctors, under a variety of brand names, as a natural infection-fighting agent. But it fell out of widespread usage after the advent of prescription antibiotics in the 1940's. Then, in the mid-1970's it experienced a dramatic resurgence in popularity after doctors discovered that many pathogens were developing immunity to prescription antibiotics. According to science writer Jim Powell in the March 1978 issue of Science Digest, "Thanks to eye-opening research, silver is re-emerging as a wonder of modern medicine. An antibiotic kills perhaps a half-dozen different disease organisms, but silver kills some 650. Resistant strains fail to develop. Moreover, silver is virtually non-toxic."

In the 1980's Dr. Robert O. Becker, MD, noted bio-medical researcher from Syracuse Medical University, and author of the best-selling book The Body Electric, discovered a distinct correlation between low silver levels in the body, and sickness. He wrote that silver deficiency is often responsible for the improper functioning of the immune system. Regarding the profound ability of metallic silver to control infection, Dr. Becker said, "All of the organisms that we tested were sensitive to the electrically generated silver ion, including some that were resistant to all known antibiotics." Regarding the safety of silver, he said, "In no case were any undesirable side effects of the silver treatment apparent."

Dr. Becker had simply re-discovered what had been known since the early 1900's. Indeed, back in 1919, Alfred Searle, founder of the Searle Pharmaceuticals firm, had written, "Applying colloidal silver to human subjects has been done in a large number of cases with astonishingly successful results... it has the advantage of being rapidly fatal to parasites without toxic action on its host. It is ?uite stable. It protects rabbits from ten times the lethal dose of tetanus or diphtheria toxin."

**How Does It Work?**- Scientists say colloidal silver works in three powerful ways: First, it works as a catalyst, disabling the enzyme that single-celled bacteria, fungi and viruses use for respiration and metabolism. Second, much like iron, it is a powerful carrier of oxygen. When it comes into contact with an infectious microbe, it releases an oxygen "burst" much like hydrogen peroxide, which kills the pathogen. Third, brand new research has shown that in tougher cases such as viral infections, the tiny silver particles simply attach to the DNA of the virus and prevent it from replicating. No replication means no further spread of infection!

Unlike antibiotics, resistant strains have never been known to develop to silver. In fact, experts say that very few disease-causing microbes tested have been able to live in the presence of even minute traces of silver for very long.

**What Can Colloidal Silver Be Used On?** -Here is a short list of diseases against which colloidal silver has been used successfully, according to historical medical texts: acne, allergies, appendicitis, arthritis, bubonic plague, burns (topical silver is one of the few treatments that can keep severe burn patients alive), cancer, candida albicans, cholera, chronic fatigue, colds and flu, Pink Eye, sties and other eye infections, diabetes, gonorrhea, hay fever, herpes, leprosy, leukemia, lupus, lymphangitis, Lyme disease, malaria, meningitis, pneumonia, rheumatism, ringworm, scarlet fever, infections of the ears, mouth and throat, shingles, skin cancer, staph infections, strep infections, syphilis, toxemia, trenchfoot, certain viruses, warts and stomach ulcers.

**On Vacation?**- Colloidal silver can also be used to purify drinking water. Most experts recommend adding one or two ounces of colloidal silver per gallon to keep drinking water germ-free. Experts also say colloidal silver used internally is one of the best antidotes for food poisoning. Some researchers suggest taking one ounce every 10 minutes throughout the day until symptoms subside. Don't go on vacation without it!

**How Is It Used?**-- Colloidal silver is most often ingested orally, but it can also be sprayed externally onto cuts or burns to prevent infection and accelerate healing. Millions of Americans drink anywhere from a tablespoon to an ounce each morning as a daily mineral supplement, to help build immunity and prevent infection. Others use it only when they are sick. People have been known to take as many as four to 12 ounces a day, or sometimes even more. Users say it will generally clear up a mild to moderate infection in only a few days, while more serious infections may take longer. (Always consult with a licensed health care practitioner for serious health conditions.)

**Where Can It Be Found?**Colloidal silver is widely available through health food stores or on the internet. There are literally thousands of vendors across the United States and Canada, offering a variety of colloidal silver products for about $30 for a tiny four-ounce bottle. That's a little expensive. Fortunately, you don't have to spend a lot of money to enjoy the phenomenal healing benefits of colloidal silver. Why? Because you can very easily make your own high-?uality colloidal silver, at home, for about thirty six cents per quart, using a safe, simple electronic device called a colloidal silver generator.

# THREE

## SOME COMMON APPLICATIONS

Colloidal silver is basically a liquid suspension composed of microscopic silver particles. Despite the fact that silver has been used for various re?uirements through the entire history of mankind, over the last few years science has identified many new uses for this.

In ancient times, when individuals first commenced to utilize silver for health reasons, it was basically used for the preservation of essential fluids like wine and milk, which very likely helps to explain why people in the modern era still use some sort of it for similar reasons. At some point in time, people even put silver into bottles of milk to keep it from going bad for a longer time. Colloidal silver, even today, can be utilized with water in much the same way.

An additional medical utilization of colloidal silver may be for treating burns. The substance contains the potential to cure burns without leaving behind a scar. Colloidal silver does not have any adverse reactions whatsoever when used for the objective of curing burns.One of the most crucial concepts of medicine is that sensitive traumas, particularly those which are open, need to be kept thoroughly clean and free of germs. This is the reason that medical professionals have been looking for the greatest ways to maintain germ-free surroundings for a long time. Even before the first anti-bacterial solutions were obtainable or invented, cleansing substances similar to it have been used to bring about this precondition of medical treatment.

Colloidal silver is also sprayed on garbage as well as other waste material. Using the substance properly decreases the unpleasant scent from such rotting objects. It can also ade?uately remove elements like salmonella and E. Coli bacteria from cooking area sponges and towels. For this reason this will assist in preventing food poisoning and gastrointestinal infection. The substance may also be included with meals which are canned or bottled for the objective of storage. This will keep bacteria out and maintain the food stuff healthy and nutritious for an extended period of time. In the same way it is integrated to milk and juices as it helps reduce fermentation and clabbering over a certain time frame.

In some ways colloidal silver can be utilized much in the same way as peroxide. This simply means you will be able to apply it on acne and zits on your face. People suffering from athlete's foot can benefit by colloidal silver. Spraying the interiors of your shoes when using the substance will help slow the spread of fungi. The substance also offers the potential to battle dandruff and reduce rashes on the skin. Colloidal silver is a substance that needs to be exploited by humankind. It is unfortunate that only a restricted number of individuals are presently informed of how much it can help their everyday lives, from being a superb supplement to the bathroom goods used for day-to-day hygiene to being a staple in the medicine cabinet for conditions like a sore throat.

When employed as a remedy to protect against colds and flu it could greatly decrease recovery time. It works much the same way for other sicknesses such as pneumonia and different respiratory infections. Doctors have even utilized colloidal silver to cure eye diseases. One must always know that the precise volume of this silver that is to be used for each goal differs. Hence one ought to not experiment with the substance on one's own rather than obtaining expert assistance.

# FOUR

# How Can it Help You?

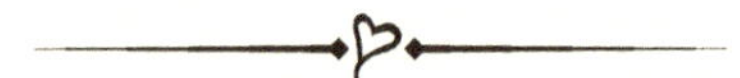

Silver is one of the most universal antibiotic substances. When administered in the colloidal form, it is for all practical purposes, non-toxic. Silver has been proven to be useful against hundreds of infectious conditions. Although the exact mechanism for the proven antimicrobial effects of colloidal silver is unknown, the most accepted theory is that colloidal silver disables the specific enzyme that many forms of bacteria, viruses and fungi utilize for their metabolism.

Colloidal silver is the result of an electromagnetic process that pulls microscopic particles from a larger piece of silver into a li?uid, such as water. These microscopic particles can more easily penetrate and travel throughout the body. Colloidal works as a catalyst, disabling the enzyme that all one-celled bacteria fungi and viruses use for their oxygen metabolism. In short, the bad guys suffocate. Unlike with antibiotics, resistant strains have never been known to develop. In fact, antibiotics are only effective against perhaps a dozen forms of bacteria and fungi, but never viruses.

Because no known disease-causing organism can live in the presence of even minute traces of chemical element metallic silver, colloidal silver is effective against more than 650 different disease-causing pathogens.

The above discussed anti bacterial properties of colloidal silver was found by scientists in early 1900's. However, discovery of antibiotics led to almost erosion of colloidal silver. The comeback of colloidal silver in medicine began in the 1970's. The late Dr. Carl Moyer, chairman of Washington University's Department of Surgery, received a grant to develop better treatments for burn victims. Dr. Margraf, the chief biochemist, worked with Dr. Moyer and other surgeons to find an antiseptic strong enough, yet safe enough, to use over large areas of the body. As a result of their efforts, and that of other researchers, hundreds of important new medical uses for silver were found. Another fact favoring colloidal silver has been the recent revolution in the technology of colloidal silver production. It is possible now to produce far more superior silver colloids such as Sovereign Silver, at a far more reasonable cost than previously possible. This revolution in silver colloid could well see science go full circle, as antibiotics become more and more out of reach and unable to cope with the new range of super bugs such as MRSA that are sweeping the globe and eventually being replaced by their own predecessor, silver colloid.

The future of colloidal silver is bright. Hopefully with today's technological advances, we can avoid the past mistakes and benefit from its wide range of advantages to prevent and treat infectious disorders. Although reports on the use of colloidal silver have spanned the past 100 years, research relating to its recent use is limited. However, through a growing number of physicians, dentists, veterinarians, nutritionists and satisfied users, information regarding the modern day uses of colloidal silver is mounting.

One of the areas of interest has been relevance of colloidal silver in treatment of AIDS. In a groundbreaking study, the Journal of Nanotechnology has published a study that found silver nanoparticles kills HIV-1 and is likely to kill virtually any other virus. An obscure but crucial discovery was made at the Biochemistry Unit of Upjohn Laboratories in 1991. Among a number of metal ions tested, Zn2+ (zinc), Cn2+ (copper), and Ag1+ (silver) were found to be the most effective inhibitors of renin and the HIV protease. This was the first report that silver is a highly effective protease inhibitor. Over the following years, this same discovery would be made several times. A year later, this same discovery was made at the University Medical Center in Geneva, Switzerland. As per him, Metal-binding proteins are important components of retroviruses such as human immunodeficiency virus (HIV). Therefore, metals could be used as antiviral agents. Silver is a highly active bactericidal metal with little toxicity for humans. These findings have opened an important avenue for research. A lot of research is being conducted in this direction and though a concrete result is not yet available, hopefully in near future, colloidal silver may prove to be an essential part in treatment of AIDS.

Colloidal silver will also be used extensively in skin care industry in coming years. More and more people are accepting the virtues of colloidal silver and its usefulness for healthy skin. It has opened doors for usage of colloidal silver in cosmetic products. The cosmetic industry is growing at fast pace and it is quite appropriate time for colloidal silver to be part of it. Colloidal silver has been already used as a main ingredient in soap manufacturing, which has proven to be a big success. The colloidal silver soap has proven itself in curing various skin disorders like acne, skin rashes, athlete's foot etc. It has also been found as rejuvenating to the human skin. It is also being used in lotion, shampoo etc. In coming years, it may find its usage in other household products as well.

Scientists are also experimenting about the use of colloidal silver in the field of treatment of deadly diseases like cancer etc. The way things are progressing, it can be said that the days are not far when colloidal silver may prove to be a cure for cancer too.

Overall, it seems that the effective and safe use of colloidal silver in the treatment of dozens of common infectious disorders is only limited by the imagination and creativity of those afflicted.

# FIVE

## COMMON USES

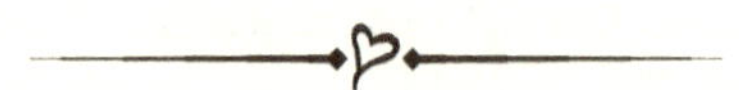

The term "colloidal silver" covers a diverse range of related products that have been in use as anti-microbial agents since at least the late 1800's. Some were produced by electrolysis and some were produced chemically. It remained in use as the primary such product until about 1938 when penicillin was developed as a more economical method of fighting germs in the human body. Since its initial development, colloidal silver has been primarily silver particles suspended in water.

The definition of the word "colloid" has two distinct meanings that should be remembered. The Chemistry definition of "colloid" is, "a system in which finely divided particles are dispersed within a continuous medium (such as water) in a manner that prevents them from being easily filtered or rapidly settled."

There are also Physiology and Pathology definitions of "colloid" from that have a completely different and unrelated meanings to the Chemistry definition. The Physiology definition is, "the gelatinous product of the thyroid gland, consisting mainly of thyroglobulin, which serves as the precursor and storage form of thyroid hormone." The Pathology definition is, "a gelatinous material resulting from colloid degeneration in diseased tissue."

The word "colloid/colloidal" may be used to refer to both gelatinous and non-gelatinous based products. The Chemistry definition could be applied to both kinds of products, but using the Physiology and Pathology definitions could only be generally applied to gelatinous/protein based products and even that is a stretch unless you ignore the fact that they are specifically referencing product of the thyroid gland and diseased tissue.

The only known potential negative side effect of "colloidal silver" has been that with heavy and prolonged use of gelatinous based silver products, a cosmetic condition called Argyria may develop. According to the World Health Organization (WHO 1993) and the United States Environmental Protection Agency silver poses no toxic effect and that extreme overuse may cause this cosmetic condition. (USEPA 1992, 2001) It is believed that these gelatins/proteins greatly increase the chance that silver may be deposited under the epidermal layer of the skin. Imagine placing a handful of BBs or marbles in a bowl of water; they will immediately sink to the bottom of the bowl. ...But if you place those same objects in a bowl of Jell-o, they will not sink to the bottom as readily.

These gelatinous additives are only re?uired where the silver particle size is too large to stay suspended in only water. One of the primary silver sources has been silver nitrate, which tends to be comprised of very large silver particles, hence the need for a gelatin base to keep it suspended. With methods utilizing some of the original, but improved, electrolysis principles, it is no longer necessary to use gelantinous or protein bases to keep the silver particles suspended. If the silver particle size is small enough, they will stay suspended by Brownian Motion indefinitely in simply deionized/distilled water, greatly reducing or eliminating most concerns of developing Argyria. This doesn't mean that it is OK to drink large quantities of silver and water for prolonged periods; there may well be some level of too much silver, but it is unknown. Every consumable food, drink, supplement and drug probably has some level where it may cause adverse effects. A few aspirin will relieve a headache, but consuming a bottle can cause death.

Although silver is found throughout nature, its occurrence is still rare enough to give it semi-precious value. Silver is the most chemically active of the "noble" metals and is harder than gold but softer than copper. It is usually stable in pure air and water but tarnishes when exposed to sulfur, hydrogen sulfide or ozone. Because of its softness and known health properties silver was used for food and drink vessels, jewelry and as a medium of monetary exchange. Evidence of silver mining has been found in Asia Minor and the Aegean Sea area as far back as 3000-4000 years B.C.

# SIX

## TREATMENT OF SKIN RASH

Skin rash or body rash is usually an inflammation on the skin. It results in change in color and texture of the affected area. Skin or body rash could be the result of irritation, disease or an allergic reaction. Allergies could be to food, plants, chemicals, animals, insects or other environmental factors. This kind of skin rash could affect the entire body or be area specific. Eruptions on the skin of the back are called Back Rash. Though not all body rashes are contagious, some could be.

The symptoms of skin rash include little, red itchy or non-itchy bumps on the skin. The affected person also feels a stinging or burning sensation on the affected area. Sometimes skin may get cracked or blistered.

Skin rash could occur as a result of a variety of reasons. Consequently, its treatment too varies widely depending on its causes. Diagnosis must take into account such things as the appearance of the rash, other symptoms, what the patient may have been exposed to, occupation, and occurrence in family members. Therefore, it is of utmost importance to decide what category the rash falls into.

Scaly, itchy skin patches usually represent one of the skin rash conditions referred to as eczema. Atopic dermatitis is perhaps the most common form of eczema. This is a hereditary skin problem that often begins in childhood as chapped cheeks and scaly patches on the scalp, arms, legs, and torso. In atopic dermatitis, the skin becomes extremely itchy and inflamed, causing redness, swelling, cracking, weeping, crusting, and scaling.

Contact dermatitis is an often-misused term which refers to a rash brought on by contact with a specific material which cause allergy on the skin. Common examples are poison ivy and reactions to costume jewelry containing nickel. Contact dermatitis affects just those parts of the skin touched by whatever material causes the allergy.

When infections appear as rashes, the most common culprits are fungi or bacterial infections. Fungal infections have nothing to do with hygiene as clean people get them too. Despite their reputation, fungal rashes are not commonly caught from dogs or other animals, nor are they easily transmitted in gyms, showers, pools, or locker rooms. In most cases they are not highly contagious between people either. In the category of skin rashes caused by bacterial infection, impetigo is the most common name. Impetigo is caused by staph or strep germs and is much more common in children than adults.

Viral rash is another variety of skin rash caused by viral infections. Viral rashes are more often symmetrical and everywhere in body. Patients with such rashes may or may not have other viral symptoms like coughing, sneezing or a stomach upset. Viral rashes usually last a few days to a week and go way on their own.

Skin rash is very common and emotionally damaging. The sad part is that people do not realize that it can be treated easily. In case of skin rashes not caused by infections, it is best to avoid the specific cause, like the allergy causing material. However, the most skin rashes are caused by bacterial infection in skins oil glands. This may happen often due to an overproduction of oils during a hormonal imbalance. Therefore, its treatment re?uires something which can penetrate and kill the bacteria. There are many medicines that may work but some cause more damage than good.

Colloidal silver is the all natural, safe and inexpensive solution for the treatment of skin rashes. It acts as a local antibiotic and also a powerful anti-inflammatory agent. It thus kills the bacteria causing the problem and also eliminates the red, itching inflammatory response! Colloidal silver has proven itself useful against all species of fungi, parasites, bacteria, protozoa, and certain viruses. Colloidal silver is the only form of silver that can be used safely as a supplement. It is absorbed into the tissues at a slow enough rate that is non irritating to the tissues. Unlike antiseptics, it does not destroy tissue cells.

Off late, the above properties of colloidal silver have been incorporated in soap manufacturing to good use. E?uipped with antimicrobial properties of colloidal silver, these soaps work wonder on several skin conditions, particularly on skin rashes. Most skin rashes respond quickly to good grades of colloidal silver, as it has not only both strong antibacterial and antiviral actions but also is an immunosupressor for many conditions. The common form of skin rashes, like poison ivy, oak and sumac all evoke an immune system over reaction, with skin irritation, itching and often blisters or oozing sores. Regular use of soap containing colloidal silver promptly stops these reactions, for blessed relief. The same usually occurs with other skin rashes.

Rashes, including blistering types, are fre?uently due to what we put on our skin. One cause is soap because it may contain an artificial chemical that produces an adverse reaction. If you have a rash problem, it is advisable to use the type of soap that is 100 percent natural or at least one that is unscented. A rash can be cleaned with a mixture composed primarily of aloe vera, along with colloidal silver, bee propolis, pau d'arco, and purified water. Then, wrap the area with gauze that is kept somewhat moist, so the mixture remains on the rash. After four or five hours, the rash should begin to heal.

It is worthwhile mentioning that any external infection of skin takes a very long time to wipe out, although it may appear to be healed in days! Internally, the blood vessels and lymph system bath each cell every few minutes but externally bacteria have many unreachable hiding spots in skins layers, hair follicles and pores, plus they may be on pillow or clothes and thus infect again as often is the case. Further, a skin rash or eruptions may result in deep tissue damage, which will take time to repair, since human skin cells live about 35 days before replacement.

A soap containing colloidal silver can penetrate skin tissues and kill off most bacteria or stop an immune system reaction, but this soap must be used regularly, even though the skin looks great in a few days.

# SEVEN

## PURCHASE AND PRODUCTION

Not all brands of Colloidal Silver are e?ual or of the same ?uality. Select a brand which is produced by the electro-colloidal, non-chemical method.

- Look at the ingredients to see it contains only silver and de-mineralized or distilled water. If the ingredients include a stabilizer or any other trace elements, it might be a good idea to research this product well.

- If it is suggested that the Colloidal Silver be refrigerated, this is an indication of another element present that could spoil. Colloidal Silver needs no refrigeration and should always be protected from freezing.

- The ideal color of Colloidal Silver should be a golden yellow, unless it is produced in concentrated form to be diluted, in which case it may be a dense looking greenish gray with an orange cast in the light. (Concentrated Colloidal Silver should return to the clear, golden yellow after dilution) A darker color could indicate larger particles of silver, or that the water used contains minerals... so check the product out.

- Colloidal Silver should be packaged in amber or cobalt blue glass, and the product should be stored in a cool dark place.

- Question the product if the directions state: 'shake well before using'. Colloidal Silver should not be shaken or stirred.

Colloidal Silver is sold and packaged in a variety of ways. There are sprays and misters; nasal sprayers and droppers; salves and compress solutions.

Colloidal Silver- Particle Surface Area: Other factors to consider when researching a Colloidal Silver product are: Particle Size and Particle Surface Area, if the information is available. Colloidal Silver products which are actually compounds do not accurately reflect the amount of Silver in the product. Also, it is the surface area of the Silver that must be exposed to the bacteria or microbe, and proteins or salts attached to the Silver particle actually block the Silver from it's environment.

So, Particle size is extremely important, but for a reason you may not expect. When it comes to Colloidal Silver, the smaller the particle the better.

Typically, manufacturers of Colloidal Silver list the Silver concentration in ppm's- parts per million. This measurment actually refers to weight; the weight of 1 part silver to a million parts water. If the particles are large, the surface area is actually smaller than if that particle were broken down to smaller particles. Picture a Rubik's Cube. In one piece it has a definite surface area; but take it apart and measure the surface area of the smaller parts; break those down again and so on... and the surface area is multiplied exponentially.

Colloidal Silver Production at Home: There is good reason to purchase a generator and produce your own Colloidal Silver at home. You can control the ?uality and the price. Colloidal Silver can be made at home for the cost of distilled water and your time. These days Colloidal Silver Generators practically run themselves once they are turned on and will turn themselves off, so your time may not be a factor. There are other generators which may require constant attendance to change the voltage polarity every couple minutes when producing concentrated Colloidal Silver to be diluted into large volumes.

If you have decided you are going to produce your own Colloidal Silver at home, there are some things to consider. If you want to produce good Colloidal Silver, a suggestion is to choose a system that uses silver rods and distilled water as the only ingredients.

You will want to use high quality distilled water in producing the Colloidal Silver. Not tap water, well water, mineral water, purified water or de-ionized water. These waters all have too many chemicals and minerals in them and de-ionized water is not sufficiently conductive. The water is very important if you want control over your production. Choosing your brand of distilled water can sometimes be a gamble. A good rule of thumb: don't buy the cheapest. You may also have to experiment with brands of distilled water. If your Colloidal Silver turns grey or brownish, the distilled water has too many minerals remaining and will not do. If this happens, you should start over with your production.

If the generator manufacturer suggests adding salt during the process to increase electrical conductivity and lessen production time, be warned that you will be producing a silver compound and not pure Colloidal Silver. Silver Chloride will always form in the presence of any salt. Also, by speeding up the production time with salt, you risk having silver particles that are too large to remain suspended in the water for very long and the silver particles will settle to the bottom of the container. It also takes longer for compounds to pass through the body.

As a sidenote... a typical suggested dose for Colloidal Silver is a teaspoon a day. This topic will not be dealt with here, because that is up to the individual. But start out with a low dose to keep the body from detoxing too ?uickly. Once the Silver goes to work and the body starts dumping the toxins into the bloodstream to be eliminated, you might actually begin to feel under the weather if you ingest larger ?uantities. If you are sick at the time of starting to take Colloidal Silver, you still want to keep your consumption rate reasonable.

# Disclaimer

**Introduction**

By using this book, you accept this disclaimer in full.

**No advice**

The book contains information. The information is not advice and should not be treated as such.

**No representations or warranties**

To the maximum extent permitted by applicable law and subject to section below, we exclude all representations, warranties, undertakings and guarantees relating to the book.

Without prejudice to the generality of the foregoing paragraph, we do not represent, warrant, undertake or guarantee:

- that the information in the book is correct, accurate, complete or non-misleading.

- that the use of the guidance in the book will lead to any particular outcome or result.

**Limitations and exclusions of liability**

The limitations and exclusions of liability set out in this section and elsewhere in this disclaimer: are subject to section 6 below; and govern all liabilities arising under the disclaimer or in relation to the book, including liabilities arising in contract, in tort (including negligence) and for breach of statutory duty.

We will not be liable to you in respect of any losses arising out of any event or events beyond our reasonable control.

We will not be liable to you in respect of any business losses, including without limitation loss of or damage to profits, income, revenue, use, production, anticipated savings, business, contracts, commercial opportunities or goodwill.

We will not be liable to you in respect of any loss or corruption of any data, database or software.

We will not be liable to you in respect of any special, indirect or consequential loss or damage.

**Exceptions**

Nothing in this disclaimer shall: limit or exclude our liability for death or personal injury resulting from negligence; limit or exclude our liability for fraud or fraudulent misrepresentation; limit any of our liabilities in any way that is not permitted under applicable law; or exclude any of our liabilities that may not be excluded under applicable law.

**Severability**

If a section of this disclaimer is determined by any court or other competent authority to be unlawful and/or unenforceable, the other sections of this disclaimer continue in effect.

If any unlawful and/or unenforceable section would be lawful or enforceable if part of it were deleted, that part will be deemed to be deleted, and the rest of the section will continue in effect.

**Law and jurisdiction**

This disclaimer will be governed by and construed in accordance with Swiss law, and any disputes relating to this disclaimer will be subject to the exclusive jurisdiction of the courts of Switzerland.